Divine Healing

DIVINE HEALING

The Origin and Cure of Disease

As Taught in the Bible
and Explained by

EMANUEL SWEDENBORG

With an Introduction by

CLYDE W. BROOMELL

"It is the spirit that quickeneth; the flesh profiteth nothing: the words that I speak unto you, they are spirit, and they are life."—*St. John* vi. 63.

"By peace, the Ancients meant in the supreme sense the Lord Himself; in the internal sense, His kingdom, and life in Him or salvation; but in the external sense, safety in the world, or health."—SWEDENBORG, *Arcana*, 4681.

BOSTON
GEO. H. ELLIS CO., PRINTERS, 272 CONGRESS STREET
1907

CONTENTS

FOREWORD

Truth needs no defence, it is its own power and explanation. Truth is not a mere statement of words, it is the consciously perceived activity of God's love and wisdom in the plane of the human mind. We advance, therefore, by the affirmation, "yea, yea," of good and the negation, "nay, nay," of evil.

This brief compilation of statements from the voluminous works of Swedenborg comes forth to meet the cry—"What portion of Truth lies back of those systems claiming the power of Divine Healing?"

No attempt is made to analyse the intellectual concepts of popular systems, such as "New-Thought," "Mental Healing," "Christian Science," and other forms of Psychopathy. If there is error in their *explanation* of the Law, we shall be of small service in beholding the "mote," merely, and calling attention to it, before we have considered the "beam" in our own eye. Trees are judged by their fruits; the good which they inaugurate comes forth by another and immutable law whereby life flows into that mind which affirms and seeks good.

It is hoped that those who read these pages will find reason for that broader charity, first enunciated by our Lord,—"he that is not against us is on our part."

As an indication of Swedenborg's entire system, even upon the one subject of the relation of soul and body, this compilation is too fragmentary and exclusive. But those who are familiar with modern thought cannot fail to see that the true philosophy of how the Divine life restores and heals humanity was more fully set forth by Swedenborg, long before the partial and limited teachings of to-day were conceived.

Students who seek a fuller knowledge of Divine order, of which health is an effect, will find ample reward in the teachings concerning Degrees, Influx, Correspondences, Soul, Body, and related subjects.

I

INTRODUCTION

The questions concerning life and death, health and disease, have been and ever will be of all-absorbing interest;—because, "All that a man hath will he give for his life."

With this new period of the world's life comes the reawakening of humanity to its birth-right of spiritual, intellectual, moral and civil order; this needs no other demonstration than "the signs following." Life is inflowing, we are feeling it; light is breaking through the clouds, men are working in it,—working to such good advantage that we say, "This is a New Age." But the startling activity comes from the same fundamental principles which have generated the good things throughout human history.

True philosophy and theology have always taught the Unity of life, the subsistence of the creature from the constant expression of the Divine. Swedenborg has not added to this general idea, it was not necessary; but he has given it new meaning and force. He has broken the shell of the general concept and brought to light the complex but most orderly arrangement of all that lies within the totality of human experience.

No one can become aware of the purport of Swedenborg's teaching of discrete degrees, the Maximus Homo or Greatest Man of the Spiritual heavens—as well as of the starry heavens with their spiritual and natural influences, and the correspondence or cause and effect

relation now and forever existing between God, the
heavens, man, and the lower orders of creation, without
entering into both the knowledge of Divine order and the
power to bring all things, even to the physical body, into
order, harmony and consequent health and use.

The Transfiguration of the Lord upon the Mount was
no mere symbol with only historic significance. The in-
dwelling of love in the will, of truth in the understanding,
and the exercise of charity in a life of use, represented
by the Disciples John, Peter and James, now, as then,
will lift any man to the summit of ideal conceptions of
humanity.

When our intellectual ideas are buried and resurrected
in true Religion, which is the totality of feeling or consciousness of the reality of the Divine and supernatural,
together with a realization of absolute and momentary
dependence upon the Divine, we shall have the faith
that removes all "mountains" or obstructions.

There is no sickness which does not originate in the
lusts of some person's will acting through falsities in his
understanding. The demoniac boy, whom the Lord
healed when He came down from the Mount of Transfiguration, is the type of all who are in the "fire" of lust
and the "water" of false imaginations. There are but
two phases in our preparation to become embodiments
and transmitters of the inflowing, healing life from the
Lord,—namely, "fasting and prayer": In terms of experience, all gratifications of the natural man are to be
eliminated, in so far as they are indulged as ends in themselves; and all power is to be gained by constant, una-
bated turning of mind and heart to the Lord in His Omnipotence, Omniscience and Omnipresence.

The power of thought is just beginning to be tested; as the means to Divine and orderly ends there is nothing that it cannot do. When Moses held aloft the brazen serpent, it was a sign to those who had been poisoned, that the only cure was to elevate the sensual man to his proper place. This could be done by constant turning of the thought to the Divine, that life might come in and eliminate death. When the Lord lifted up His Humanity, it was that we might also have a constant standard toward which to direct the thoughts, and in that attitude become recipients of a heavenly influx.

There is nothing miraculous, in the vulgar sense, about the cures effected through faith. Ignorance of the law involved causes wonder, sometimes doubt and rejection. It is not the mere belief or thought which is the salvation and cure; the thought is but the means, while salvation is the effect. The solution is here: Just as a current of electricity can flow only along the lines of a *connected* circuit, so the life-force can flow through the human mind only in the direction of *unbroken* thought,—the thought which indicates the secret ends and purposes of the life's ruling love.

This may be made clearer by another form of illustration: Man is an organized spiritual being who possesses a material body. The body lives from the soul; the soul lives from God. The will and its loves, the understanding and its thoughts constitute the regnant principles of the soul. The heart and lungs reign universally in the body, but the quality of life imparted to the various organs is determined by the influx of the soul's life from the will into the heart, and from the understanding into the lungs. That the heart and lungs correspond immediately to the reigning loves and thoughts of the soul needs no further proof than the most common reflection upon the changes in action of these two organs, when the feelings and thoughts are passing through marked states.

A change in the totality of consciousness means a like change in the physical organism. Do we fail in our attempts to have a sound mind in a sound body? It is because the thought of the Divine power and presence is transient and spasmodic, when it should be the sign of the life-stream's direction.

When once the fundamental laws of our being are understood and embodied, the effort of one man to cure another will be a normal condition. There can be no help in merely making a verbal contradiction of another man's disease. But the spoken word of truth will awaken the sickened mind of another, while the sphere of a heart overflowing with tender sympathy will penetrate both body and soul of the needy one. This sphere, in a highly developed state, can be extended and directed voluntarily, upon the same principle that the Lord is omnipresent, and that the angels nearest to Him in quality of life have a sphere which extends to the boundaries of heaven. Thought filled with love is quite enough to touch those who are already sensitive to spiritual influence; but where the disease has deadened the sensibilities of both soul and body, the life sphere must frequently be conveyed by the hand; for in the hand the whole nature of a man is ultimated.

To bring the subject to a practical issue: There is much in the illogical, unphilosophical statements of certain modern schools of mental healing which seems to act as a stumbling-block to those seeking light and life. However, it is not what we call things, but the use we make of them that determines results; it is not the pseudo-philosophical falsity of ignorance, but the constant affirmation of the positive and known good which produces the salutary effect.

There are those who admit the propriety of Divine healing as a thing useful in former ages and as something quite probable in times to come. They are well grounded in doctrines *about* order, influx, and correspondence; but here they rest like the impotent man upon his bed. Continuous thought upon the Lord's question "Whether it is easier to say, thy sins be forgiven thee, or take up thy bed and walk" does not occur to these partial believers. It would be a startling discovery to those who swallow Swedenborg whole, but never digest his system in detail, and who argue that sickness of body is not incompatible with health of soul, if they should realize the full meaning of both the Bible's and Swedenborg's teaching on the matter. In Divine Providence, No. 142, it is stated that "no one is reformed in a state of sickness, because reason is not then in a free state; for the state of the mind depends upon the state of the body. When the body is sick, the mind also is sick."

It quite often happens that a sphere of humility and goodness pervades the chamber of a sick person; but here again the teaching of Swedenborg and the Bible are in accord. The Bible would teach that the mind was weak and diseased, else it would affect its body with health; Swedenborg teaches that sicknesses, griefs, and misfortunes break the lusts and desires of the self-life and hold the man in a state of humility and acknowledgment of the Divine, but that reformation and advance cannot take place until the body and mind are well and act in correspondence, or else are severed so that the man enters a state of instruction in the spiritual world.

A sound mind in a sound body is the true order of man. Sin, or, what is better understood, all the elements of selfishness are the primal causes of disease of mind and body. If disease is contagious and may be absorbed by the guiltless, so health is more contagious and may be absorbed by the guilty. That we may receive and transmit life should be our ruling desire. The "tree of life" is in the midst of every soul, though the false conceptions of life, springing from placing the senses above the spirit, may seem to remove it to the borders or background of consciousness. When we take our knowledge of the Lord's Omniscience, Omnipresence and Omnipotence as a fact for conscious experience, when we believe influx to be not a theory, but our life, when the *facts* of correspondence of soul and body are employed in place of the *theory*, then again will the "tree of life" appear in the centre of consciousness, growing, not without our care, as in the Eden-Garden of childlike delight, but, springing from the thought-ways of an orderly and well-used mind, it will produce the fruit of all manner of spiritual satisfactions and will scatter itself abroad like leaves for the healing of nations, producing the universal "peace of God,"—the New Jerusalem.

CLYDE W. BROOMELL.

Boston, 1907.

II

SOUL AND BODY

The soul, in a proper sense, signifies that in man which lives; consequently his life itself. That in man which lives is not the body, but the soul, and by the soul the body lives. The life of man, or his living principle, is derived from celestial love, and nothing living can possibly exist which has not thence its origin.—HEAVENLY ARCANA, 1436.

The term soul, as used in the Word, signifies in a universal sense all life; for soul in a universal sense is that by and from which another thing is and lives, thus the soul of the body is its spirit; for by and from the spirit the body lives; but the soul of the spirit is its life still more interior, by and from which it has wisdom and intelligence.—HEAVENLY ARCANA, 2930.

Every man has an internal and an external, for the internal is his thought and his will, and the external is his speech and his action. With those who are in the good of love and the truths of faith, the internal man is open, and by it they are in heaven; but with those who are in evils and the falses thence derived, the internal man is closed, and by the external they are only in the world; these are they of whom it is said that they are in externals without an internal. These indeed have also interiors, but the interiors appertaining to them are the interiors of their external man, which is in the world, but not the interiors of the internal man which is in heaven; those interiors, namely, which are of the external man, when the internal is closed, are evil, yea, filthy, for they think only of the world and of themselves, and will only those things which are of the world and which are of self, and think nothing at all about heaven

Jesus Christ is center stage Revealing the Father & imparting Holy Spirit, oneness

what so ever a man thinks - so is he.

and about the Lord, yea, neither do they will these latter things.—HEAVENLY ARCANA, 10429.

What any one does from love, remains inscribed on his heart, for love is the fire of life, thus is the life of every one; hence such as the love is, such is the life, and such as the life is, such is the whole man as to soul and as to body.—HEAVENLY ARCANA, 10740.

The soul, of which it is said that it shall live after death, is nothing but the man himself, who lives in the body; that is, it is the interior man, who by the body acts in the world, and enables the body to live.

The commerce of the soul with the body is the communication of the spiritual things of heaven with the natural things of the world, and the communication is effected by influx, and is according to conjunction. This communication, which is effected by influx, according to conjunction, is at this day unknown, because all things are attributed to nature, and nothing is known of the spiritual, which at this day is so remote, that, when it is thought of, it appears as nothing.—HEAVENLY ARCANA, 6054, 6057.

There are two principles in the Lord, namely, love and wisdom, and those two principles proceed from Him; and inasmuch as man was created to be a likeness and image of Him, a likeness by love, and an image by wisdom, therefore with man there are created two receptacles, one for love and the other for wisdom; the receptacle of love is what is called the will, and the receptacle of wisdom is what is called the understanding: man knows that those two [receptacles] appertain to him, but he does not know that they are so conjoined as they are in the Lord, with this difference, that in the Lord they are life, but in man the receptacles of life.

The agreement of things with one another

⎯⎯⎯⟶ CORRESPONDENCE

The receptacles of love and of wisdom, first exist with man at his conception and birth; from them by a con-

Common denominator

Resemblence

The agreement of things w/ one other —

tinuous principle are brought forth and produced all things of the body from the head even to the soles of the feet; their productions are effected according to the laws of correspondence, and therefore all things of the body both internal and external are correspondences. *agreement*

The organic parts of the body produced from various complicated fibres, are effects, which cannot live, feel, and be moved from themselves, but from their origins by a continuous [principle]: to illustrate this by example; the eye does not see from itself, but by what is continuous from the understanding, for the understanding sees by the eye, and also moves the eye, determines it to objects, and gives intenseness to the sight; neither does the ear hear from itself, but by what is continuous from the understanding, for the understanding hears by the ears, and also determines them, makes them erect and attentive to sounds; nor does the tongue speak from itself, but from the thought of the understanding, for thought speaks by the tongue, and varies sounds, and exalts their measures at pleasure; in like manner the muscles, these not being moved of themselves, but from the will together with the understanding, which actuate them at their own disposal. It is evident, that there is not anything in the body which feels and is moved of itself, but from its origins, in which reside the understanding and will, consequently which are in man the receptacles of love and wisdom. These are the first forms; the organs both of sense and of motion are forms derived from them, for according to formation is effected influx, which is not given from the latter into the former, but from the former into the latter, for influx from the former into the latter is spiritual influx, and influx from the latter into the former is natural influx, which is also called physical.

Those productions are effected according to the laws of correspondence, and all things of the body, both internal and external, are correspondences. Correspondence is between what is natural and what is spiritual. When anything derived from a spiritual principle as its origin and cause becomes visible and perceptible before the senses, there is correspondence between those things. Such is the correspondence between the spiritual and natural things appertaining to man; spiritual things being all the things of his love and wisdom, consequently of his will and understanding, and natural things being all things relating to his body; these latter, inasmuch, as they have existed, and perpetually exist, that is subsist, from the former, are correspondences, and therefore act in unity, as end, cause, and effect; thus the face acts in unison with the affections of the mind, the speech with the thought, and the actions of all the members with the will.—DIVINE WISDOM, II.

Inasmuch as there is a correspondence of all things in the body, with all things of the mind in man, there is especially a correspondence with the heart and lungs, which correspondence is universal, because the heart reigns in the body throughout, and likewise the lungs. The heart and the lungs are the two fountains of all natural motions in the body, and the will and understanding are the two fountains of all spiritual activities in the same body, and the natural motions of the body must correspond to the activities of its spirit, for unless they correspond the life of the body would cease, and likewise the life of the mind [*animus*], correspondence causing both to exist and subsist.

That the heart corresponds to the will, or what is the same thing, to the love, is evident from the variations of its pulse according to affections. It beats either slowly or quickly, high or low, soft or hard, equally or unequally, differently in gladness and in sorrow, in tranquillity of mind and in anger, in intrepidity and in fear, in the heat of the body and in its cold, and variously in diseases. Inasmuch as the heart corresponds to the affections which are of the love and thence of the will, therefore the wise men of old ascribed affections to the heart, and some of them fixed on the heart as the abode of affections. It is customary in common discourse to speak of a magnanimous heart, a timid heart, a glad heart, a sorrowful heart, a soft heart, a hard heart, a great heart, a little heart, a sound heart, a broken heart, a fleshy heart, a stony heart, and to call a man fat-hearted, soft-hearted, vile-hearted, and to say of another that he has no heart, and to talk of giving a heart to act, of giving one heart, of giving a new heart, of stirring up in the heart, of receiving in the heart, of not ascending upon the heart, of being obstinate in heart, of being lifted up in heart, of being friendly in heart, hence also we speak of concord (agreement in heart), of discord (disagreement in heart), and in the Latin tongue, of *vecordia* (madness of heart), with several like expressions. In the Word also throughout, by heart is signified the will or love, by reason that the Word is written by mere correspondences.

The soul or spirit of the lungs, which is the respiration, corresponds to the understanding. It is said in the Word, that man ought to love God with the whole heart and the whole soul, by which is signified that he ought to love with all the will and all the understanding; in like manner that God will create in man a new heart and a new spirit, where by heart is signified the will, and by spirit the understanding, because when man is regenerated, he is created anew. The nostrils also, from the correspondence of respiration through them, signify perception. An intelligent man is said to be quick-scented, and a man not intelligent, of a fat and heavy nostril. The Lord breathed into the disciples, and said to them, "*receive ye the Holy Spirit*," (John xx. 22): by breathing into them was signified the intelligence which they were about to receive, and by the Holy Spirit is meant the divine wisdom, which teaches and illustrates man. This was done in order to show that the divine wisdom, which is meant by the Holy Spirit, proceeds from him. That soul and spirit are predicated of respiration, is also known from common discourse, for it is said of man, when he dies, that he emits the soul, and emits the spirit, inasmuch as he then ceases to have

animation and to breathe. Spirit, in most languages,
signifies each, both spirit in heaven and the breath of
man, likewise wind; hence comes the idea, that spirits
in the heavens are as winds, also that the souls of men
after death are as vapors, yea God Himself, because He
is called a spirit when yet God Himself is a man, in like
manner the soul of man after death, also every spirit
in the heavens.

That the lungs correspond to the understanding as
the heart does to the will, is further evident from man's
thought and speech; all thought is of the understanding,
and all speech is of the thought. A man cannot think
unless the pulmonary spirit concurs and is in concord,
wherefore when he thinks tacitly, he respires tacitly;
if he thinks deeply, he respires deeply; in like manner
if slowly, hastily, attentively, gently, earnestly, and so
forth.—DIVINE WISDOM, VI.

The entire heaven represents one man, and it is man
in form, and it is therefore called the Greatest Man.
The angelic societies, of which heaven consists, are ac-
cordingly arranged as the members, organs, and viscera
in man; so that some are in the head, some in the
breast, some in the arms, and some in each of their
particulars. The societies which are in any member
there, correspond to the like member in man. From
this correspondence man subsists; for man subsists
from no other source than from heaven.

Heaven is distinguished into two kingdoms, one of
which is called the celestial kingdom and the other the
spiritual kingdom. The correspondence of the two
kingdoms of heaven with the heart and lungs is the
general correspondence of heaven with man. There is
a more particular correspondence with each of his members, organs, and viscera. They who in the greatest
man, which is heaven, are in the head, are beyond others
in every good, being in love, peace, innocence, wisdom,
intelligence, and consequent joy and happiness. These
flow into the head and the things belonging to the head

with man, and correspond to them. They who in the
greatest man, or heaven, are in the breast, are in the
good of charity and faith, and also flow into the breast
of man, and correspond to it. They who in the greatest
man, or heaven, are in the loins and the organs there
devoted to generation, are in marriage love. They
who are in the feet, are in the lowest good of heaven.
They who are in the arms and hands, are in the power
of truth from good. They who are in the eyes, are in
understanding. They who are in the ears, are in hearing and obedience. They who are in the nostrils, are
in perception. They who are in the mouth and tongue
are in speech from understanding and perception. They
who are in the kidneys, are in truth searching, separating,
and chastising. They who are in the liver, pancreas,
and spleen, are in the various purification of good and
truth. They flow into the like things of man and correspond to them. The influx of heaven is into the
functions and uses of the members; and the uses, because they are from the spiritual world, form themselves by means of such things as are in the natural
world, and thus present themselves in effect.

By these same members, organs, and viscera, such
things are signified in the Word. Thus by head is signified intelligence and wisdom, by breast charity, by
loins marriage love, by arms and hands the power of
truth, by feet what is natural, by eyes understanding,
by nostrils perception, by ears obedience, by kidneys
the searching of truth. Hence also it is that men com-
monly say of one who is intelligent and wise, that he
has a head; of one who is kind, that he is a bosom-
friend; of one who has clear perception, that he is keen-
scented; of one who is intelligent, that he is sharp-
sighted; of one who is powerful, that he has long hands;
of one who wills from love, that it is from the heart.—
HEAVEN AND HELL, 90-97.

Common denominator
commonality
parallel
similarity

III

ORIGIN OF DISEASE

THE CORRESPONDENCE OF DISEASES WITH THE SPIRITUAL WORLD

All diseases appertaining to man have correspondence with the spiritual world; for whatever in the whole of nature has not correspondence with the spiritual world, has no existence, having no cause from which it can exist, consequently from which it can subsist. The things which are in nature, are mere effects, their causes are in the spiritual world, and the causes of those causes, which are ends, are in the interior heaven.

Diseases also have correspondence with the spiritual world, not indeed with heaven, which is the Grand Man, but with those who are in the opposite, thus with those who are in the hells. Diseases have correspondence with those who are in the hells because they correspond to the lusts and passions of the mind; these therefore are the origins of diseases. The common origins of diseases are intemperances, luxuries of various kinds, pleasures merely corporeal, also envyings, hatreds, revenges, lasciviousness, which destroy a man's interiors. When these are destroyed, the exteriors suffer, and draw him into disease, and thereby into death. That man is subject to death by reason of evils, or on account of sin, is well known in the church, thus also he is subject to diseases, for these are of death.

All the infernals induce diseases, but with a difference, because all the hells are in the lusts and concupiscences of evil. Heaven, which is the Grand Man, keeps all things in connection and safety; hell, as being in the opposite destroys and rends all things asunder; consequently if the infernals are applied, they induce diseases, and at length death. But they are not permitted to flow-in so far as into the solid parts of the body, or into the parts which constitute the viscera, organs, and members of man, but only into the lusts and falsities. When a man falls into disease, they then flow into such unclean things as appertain to the disease. That the case is thus, has been given me to know by much experience, and this so frequently and of so long continuance, as not to leave a doubt remaining; for evil spirits from such places have been often and for a long time applied to me, and according to their presence they induced pains, and also diseases: it was shown me where they were, and what was their quality, and it was also told me whence they came.

A certain spirit, who in the life of the body had been devoted to pleasures, and not willing to do good and be serviceable to any one, except for the sake of himself, was with me for some days, and appeared beneath the feet; when the sphere of his life was communicated to me, wherever he came, he inflicted some pain on the periostea and nerves there, as on the toes of the left foot; and when he was permitted to emerge, he inflicted pain on the parts where he was, especially on the periostea in the loins, also on the periostea of the breast beneath the diaphragm, and likewise on the inside of the teeth. When his sphere operated, it induced also a great oppression in the stomach.

There exhaled a troublesome heat, which was collected from various hells, arising from lusts of various kinds, as from haughtiness, lasciviousness, adulteries, hatreds, revenges, quarrels, and fightings. When this heat acted upon my body, it instantly induced disease like that of a burning fever; but when it ceased to flow-in, the disease instantly ceased. When a man falls into such disease, which he had contracted from his life, instantly an unclean sphere corresponding to the disease adjoins itself, and is present as the fomenting cause. That I might know for certain that this is the case, there were spirits from several hells present with me, who communicated the sphere of the exhalations thence arising, and as that sphere was permitted to act upon the solid parts of the body, I was seized with heaviness and pain, and even with disease corresponding thereto, which ceased in a moment, as those spirits were expelled: and lest any room should be left for doubt, this was repeated very many times.

There are also spirits who infuse unclean colds, like those of a cold fever, which also it was given me to know by repeated experience. The same spirits also induce such things as disturb the mind; they likewise induce swoonings.

There are certain spirits, who not only have reference to the most viscid things of the brain, which are its excrementitious parts, but also have the art of infecting them as it were with poisons. When such spirits flock together, they rush within the skull, and thence by continuity even to the spinal marrow. This cannot be felt by those whose interiors are not open. To me it was given manifestly to feel their influence, and also their attempt to kill me, but in vain, because I was defended by the Lord. It was their intention to take away from me every intellectual faculty: I was very sensible of their operation, and also of a pain derived from it, which nevertheless presently ceased. I afterwards conversed with them, and they were forced to confess whence they came. They stated that they lived in dark forests, where they dare not offer any violence to their companions, because in such case their companions are allowed to treat them with the utmost severity; thus they are kept in bonds. They are deformed, of a beastly countenance, and hairy. It was told me, that such were those, who in old time slew whole armies, as it is written in the Word; for they rushed into the chambers of the brain of each individual, and occasioned terror, together with such insanity that one slew another. Such at this day are kept shut up within their hell, and are not let out. They have reference also to the fatal tubercles of the head within the skull. It was said that they rush within the skull, and thence by continuity even into the spinal marrow; but it is an appearance that the spirits themselves rush in, they being carried out by a way which corresponds to those spaces in the body, which is felt as if the incursion were within. This is the effect of correspondence.

There is a certain kind of spirits, who, in consequence of their desire to have dominion, and to be the sole rulers over all others, with a view to that end excite among others enmities, hatreds, and combats. I have witnessed the combats, and have been surprised; and on my asking who they were, I was told that they are spirits of the above description, and that they excite such things in consequence of their intention to rule alone, according to the maxim, Divide and rule. It was also granted me to converse with them, and they immediately said that they governed all; but it was given me to answer them, that they were insane if they seek to establish their rule by such means. Their speech was with the rapidity of a current, because in the life of the body they had excelled in elocution. I was instructed that they are such as have reference to the thick phlegm of the brain, which by their presence they deprive of every principle of life, and induce torpor, whence come obstructions, from which arise several diseases, and also numbness. It was observed that they were totally void of conscience, and that they made human prudence and wisdom to consist in exciting enmities, hatreds, and intestine combats, for the sake of bearing rule.

Those who despise and ridicule the Word in the letter, and especially those who despise and ridicule those things of the Word which are in a deeper sense, consequently also the doctrinals which are derived from the Word, and at the same time are not principled in any love towards their neighbour, but in the love of self, have reference to the vitiated things of the blood, which pervade all the veins and arteries, and contaminate the whole mass.

When hypocrites who discourse holily concerning divine things, with an affection of love concerning the public and their neighbour, testify what is just and equitable, and still have despised those things in their hearts, and have even ridiculed them; when these, I say, have been attendant on me, and they were allowed to flow into the parts of the body to which they correspond from the apposite principle, they injected pain into the teeth, which upon their nearer approach was so severe that I could not endure it; and so far as they were removed, so far the pain ceased, which was shown repeatedly in order to remove all doubt. Among them was one whom I had known during his life in the body, on which account I conversed with him; and in proportion as he was present, so my teeth and gums were affected with pain; when he was lifted upwards to the left, a pain attacked the left jaw, and the bone of the left temple, and penetrated even to the bones of the cheek.

The most contumacious of all are those, who, during their life in the world, appeared more just than others, and were at the same time in appointments of dignity; hence from each source they derived authority and influence, and yet believed nothing, and lived the life of self-love alone, being inflamed with intestine hatred and revenge against all who did not favour them, and pay court to them, and especially against those who in any way opposed them. When they are applied to a man, they induce a great pain by weariness, which they inwardly excite and increase continually, even to the highest degree of impatience, which induces such infirmity in the mind and thence in the body, that the man can scarcely raise himself from his bed. This was shown me by the circumstance, that when they were present, I was seized with the above weakness, which left me according to the degree in which they were removed. They employed various arts of infusing weariness and consequent weakness, especially by reproofs and defamations, among themselves and their associates, whose common sphere they inject.

There are others who in the life of the body have been most filthy, their filthiness being of such a nature as cannot be mentioned. They, by their presence and influx into the solid parts of the body, induce such a weariness of life, and such a torpor in the members and joints, that the man cannot raise himself out of bed. They are most contumacious, and do not desist by punishments as other devils do. When they are driven away, it is not done suddenly, but slowly.

There were spirits attendant upon me, who induced such an oppression in the stomach, that I seemed to myself scarce able to live; the oppression was so great that with others it would have occasioned fainting; but they were removed, and then it instantly ceased. It was told me, that such spirits are those who in the life of the body have not been habituated to any employment, not even domestic, but only to pleasure; and besides they had lived in filthy ease and sluggishness, and had not taken any concern about others; they also despised faith: in a word, they were animals, not men. The sphere of such with the sick induces numbness in the members and joints.

There are in the brain viscid humours, with which is mixed somewhat spirituous or vital, which viscid humours, being there thrown out from the blood, fall first between the membranes, then between the fibres, part of them into the great ventricles in the brain. The spirits who have a corresponding reference to those viscid humours, are of such a quality, that, in consequence of a habit acquired in the life of the body, they excite scruples of conscience and insinuate them into things of no importance, whereby they aggravate the conscience of the simple; nor do they know what ought to move the conscience, for they make a matter of conscience of every thing that befalls them. Such also induce sensible anxiety into the part of the abdomen beneath the region of the diaphragm. They are also at hand in temptations, and occasion anxieties, which are sometimes intolerable. Such of them as correspond to the less vital viscid phlegm, on such occasions keep the thought inherent in those anxieties.

From experience it has been given me to learn that an inundation or flood in the spiritual sense is twofold, one being an inundation of lusts, and the other of falsities; an inundation of lusts is of the voluntary part, and is of the right side of the brain, whereas an inundation of falsities is of the intellectual part, in which is the left side of the brain. When a man who had lived in good, is remitted into his proprium, thus into the sphere of his own life, there appears as it were an inundation. When he is in that inundation he is indignant and angry, thinks restlessly, and desires vehemently, in one way when the left part of the brain is inundated, where falses are, and in another when the right is inundated, where evils are. But when a man is kept in the sphere of life which he had received from the Lord by regeneration, he is altogether out of such an inundation, and is as it were in serenity and sunshine, and in gladness and happiness, thus far from indignation, anger, restlessness, lusts, and the like.

As death comes from no other source than from sin, and sin is all that which is contrary to divine order, it is from this ground that evil closes the smallest and altogether invisible vessels [of the human body], of which the next greater vessels, which are also invisible, are composed; for the smallest and altogether invisible vessels are continued to a man's interiors: hence comes the first and inmost obstruction, and hence the first and inmost vitiation in the blood. This vitiation, when it increases, causes disease and at length death. But if a man had lived the life of good, his interiors would be open to heaven, and through heaven to the Lord: thus also the smallest and invisible vessels would be open, and the man would be without disease, and would only decrease to ultimate old age, until he became altogether an infant, but a wise one. When the body could no longer minister to its internal man, or spirit, he would pass without disease out of his terrestrial body, into a body such as the angels have, thus out of the world immediately into heaven.—HEAVENLY ARCANA, 5711-5726.

In the spiritual world diseases are evils and falses, spiritual diseases being nothing else; for evils and falses take away health from the internal man, and induce sicknesses in the mind, and at length pains; nor is any thing else signified in the Word by diseases. That in the Word physicians, the art of physic, and medicines, signify preservations from evils and falses, is manifest from the passages where they are named.—HEAVENLY ARCANA, 6504.

By diseases are signified spiritual diseases, which are evils destroying the life of the will of good, and falses destroying the life of the understanding of truth, in a word destroying the spiritual life which is of faith and charity. Natural diseases also correspond to such, for every disease in the human race is from that source, because from sin. Every disease also corresponds to its evil; because the all of the life of man is from the spiritual world; wherefore if his spiritual life sickens, evil is also thence derived into the natural life, and becomes a disease there.

Inasmuch as diseases represented the iniquities and evils of spiritual life, therefore by the diseases which the Lord healed, is signified liberation from the various kinds of evil and the false, which infested the church and the human race, and which would have induced spiritual death; for Divine miracles are distinguished from other miracles by this, that they involve and have respect to states of the church and heavenly kingdom. On this account the Lord's miracles consisted principally in the healing of diseases. This is meant by the Lord's words

to the disciples sent from John, "Tell John the things
which ye hear and see, the blind see, and the lame walk,
the lepers are cleansed, and the deaf hear, the dead rise
again, and the poor hear the gospel," Matt. xi. 4, 5.
Hence it is, that it is so often said, that the Lord healed
every disease and languor," Matt. iv. 23.—HEAVENLY
ARCANA, 8364.

Sores signifiy works grounded in the proprium, and
thence evil, because from man's proprium nothing but
evil can possibly be produced; for the proprium of
man is that into which he is born, and which he afterwards contracts by his own life; and whereas his proprium is thus from its very birth composed of mere evils,
therefore man must be as it were created anew, that is,
regenerated, in order that he may be in good, and so may
be received into heaven. When he is regenerated, then
the evils which are from the proprium are removed, and
in the place thereof are implanted goods, which is effected
by means of truths. That sores signify works which are
from man's proprium, may appear from the Word where
sores and wounds are mentioned, likewise diseases of
various kinds, as leprosies, fevers, hemorrhoids, and
several others, all which correspond to cupidities arising
from evil loves, and thence signify them.—APOCALYPSE
EXPLAINED, 962.

IV

SAVING AND HEALING FAITH

"Look unto me, and be ye saved,* all ye ends of the earth: for I am God, and there is none else."—ISAIAH xlv. 21.

The passages where faith and believing are mentioned in the gospels are the following: as in Matthew: "There came a centurion to the Lord, saying, Lord, I am not fit that thou shouldst come under my roof, but speak the Word only, and my boy shall be healed. Jesus hearing admired, and said to them that followed him, Verily, I say unto you, I have not found so great faith in Israel: and he said unto the centurion, Go thy way, and as thou hast believed, be it done unto thee; and his boy was healed in that hour" (viii. 8, 10, 13). The reason why the Lord healed this and other persons according to their faith, was, because the first and primary principle of the church then to be established was, that they should believe the Lord to be God Almighty, for without that faith no church could have been established. The Lord was the God of heaven, and God of earth, with whom there cannot be given any conjunction except by the acknowledgment of His divinity, which acknowledgment is faith.

"A woman labouring with an issue of blood, touched the hem of Jesus' garment; for she said within herself, if I may only touch the hem of His garment, I shall be healed. Jesus turning about and seeing her, said, Daughter, be of good comfort, thy faith hath made thee whole; and she was healed in that hour" (ix. 20, 21, 22). "They brought unto Him a paralytic lying upon a bed; Jesus, seeing their faith, said unto the paralytic, Be of good comfort, thy sins are remitted; arise, take

---

* The Hebrew idea and word saved (yasha) mean to be eased,—not diseased.

up thy bed, and go to thine house" (ix. 2–7; Luke
v. 19–25). "Two blind men cried, saying, Have mercy
upon us, thou Son of David: Jesus said unto them,
Believe ye that I am able to do this? They say unto
Him, Yea, Lord: then He touched their eyes, saying,
According to your faith, be it unto you; and their
eyes were opened" (ix. 27, 28, 29). By this faith,
whereby the sick were healed, is understood no other
faith than that which is called historical, which also
at that time was miraculous. The faith was, that
the Lord was Almighty, because he was able to do
miracles of Himself, wherefore also He allowed Himself to be worshipped, which was not the case with
the prophets of the Old Testament, who were not worshipped. This historical faith in all cases precedes,
before the same becomes saving. Historical faith
becomes saving with man, when he learns truths from
the Word, and lives according to them.

Again, in Matthew: "A woman of Canaan, whose
daughter was agitated by a demon, came and worshipped Jesus, saying, Lord, help me; Jesus said unto
her, Great is thy faith, be it unto thee as thou wilt:
and her daughter was healed" (xv. 22–28). In John:
"A ruler, whose son was sick, entreated Jesus that He
would heal his son before he died: Jesus said unto him,
Go thy way, thy son liveth; and the man believed in
the word which Jesus said unto him, and his servants
met him, saying, Thy son liveth; therefore he believed,
and his whole house" (iv. 46–53). "Jesus finding the
man born blind, whom He healed, said unto him, Be-
lievest thou then in the Son of God? He answered
him and said, Who is he, Lord, that I may believe in
Him? He said unto him, Thou also seest Him, and
He who speaketh with thee is He: he said, Lord, I
believe; and he worshipped Him" (ix. 35–38). In
Luke: "Jesus said to the ruler of the synagogue, whose
daughter was dead, Fear not, believe only, and she
shall be made whole; and she arose again" (viii. 50,

55). "One of the ten lepers that were healed by the Lord, who was a Samaritan, returned, and fell upon his face at the feet of Jesus; and Jesus said unto him, Arise, go thy way, thy faith hath made thee whole" (xvii. 19). "Jesus said to the blind man, Thy faith hath made thee whole; and immediately his sight was restored" (xviii. 42, 43). In Mark: "Jesus said to the father of a child who had a dumb spirit, whom his disciples could not heal, If thou canst believe, all things are possible to him that believeth. The father of the child, crying out with tears, said, Lord, I believe, help thou mine unbelief: and he was healed" (ix. 17, 23, 24).

There were three reasons why faith in the Lord healed them, the first was, their acknowledging His divine omnipotence, and that He was God; the second was, because faith is acknowledgment and from acknowledgment intuition, and all intuition from acknowledgment causes another to be present, which is a common thing in the spiritual world; the third reason was, that all the diseases which the Lord healed, represented and thence signified spiritual diseases, to which natural diseases correspond, and spiritual diseases cannot be healed except by the Lord, and indeed by looking to his divine omnipotence, and by repentance of the life, wherefore also He sometimes said, thy sins are remitted thee, go and sin no more. The faith whereby spiritual diseases are healed by the Lord, can only be given by truths from the Word, and by a life according to them, the truths themselves and the life according to them constituting the quality of the faith.

Again, in John: "The sister of Lazarus who was now dead, said to Jesus, Lord, by this time he stinketh: Jesus said unto her, Said I not unto thee, if thou wouldst believe thou shouldst see the glory of God" (xi. 39, 40). In Luke: "Jesus said to the woman who was a sinner, who made His feet wet with her tears, and wiped them with the hair of her head, and kissed His feet, which she also anointed with oil, Thy sins are

remitted thee, thy faith hath made thee whole, go in
peace" (vii. 38, 48, 50). From these words also it is
evident, that faith in the omnipotence of the Lord
healed them, and also that the same faith remitted,
that is, removed, their sins. The reason was, because
that woman not only had faith in the divine omnipotence of the Lord, but also loved Him, for she kissed
His feet, and therefore the Lord said, thy sins are remitted thee, thy faith hath made thee whole. Faith
causes the Divine [principle] of the Lord to be present,
and love conjoins, for it is possible for the Lord to be
present and not conjoined, whence it is evident that
faith derived from love is the faith which saves.

Again: "Jesus said to the disciples in the ship, Why
are ye fearful, O ye of little faith; then He arose, and
rebuked the wind and the sea, and there was a great
calm" (Matt. viii. 26; Mark iv. 39, 40, 41; Luke viii.
24, 25). "Peter, at the bidding of Jesus, descended
out of the ship, and walked upon the waters; but when
the wind became boisterous, he feared greatly, and,
beginning to sink, cried out, Lord, save me; Jesus immediately caught hold of his hand, and said, Thou
man of little faith, wherefore didst thou doubt" (Matt.
xiv. 28–31). "When the disciples could not heal the
lunatic, Jesus said unto them, O incredulous and per-
verse generation, how long shall I be with you? and
Jesus healed him; and He said to the disciples, that
they could not heal him by reason of their unbelief"
(Matthew xvii. 14). "When Jesus came into His own
country, and they were there offended in Him, He said,
A prophet is not without honour except in his own country, and in his own house; therefore He did not many
virtues there by reason of their unbelief" (Matthew
xiii. 57, 58).

The reason why the Lord called the disciples men
of little faith when they could not do miracles in His
name, and why He could not do miracles in His own
country on account of their unbelief, was, because

the disciples did indeed believe the Lord to be the Messiah or Christ, likewise the Son of God, and the prophet of whom it was written in the Word, but still they did not yet believe in Him as God omnipotent, and that Jehovah the Father was in Him. In proportion as they believed Him to be a man, and not at the same time God, His Divine [principle], to which omnipotence belonged, could not become present with them by faith. Faith causes the Lord to be present, but faith in Him as a man only, does not bring His divine omnipotence present; which also is the reason why they cannot be saved, who, at this day in the world, look unto His Human [principle] and not at the same time unto His Divine.

It was from a similar cause that the Lord could not do miracles in His own country, for they there saw Him from infancy, like another man, and therefore could not add to this idea the idea of His divinity, and when this idea is not present, the Lord is indeed present in man, but not with divine omnipotence, for faith causes the presence of the Lord in man according to the quality of the perception concerning Him. The rest man does not acknowledge and so rejects. In order to the Lord's operating anything by faith with man, the presence of His divine [principle] must be in man, and not out of him.

Again, in John: "Many of the multitude believed in Jesus, and said, when Christ shall come, will He do more signs than this man doeth" (vii. 31). In Mark: "These signs shall follow them that believe: in My name they shall cast out demons, they shall speak with new tongues, they shall take up serpents, if they drink any deadly thing it shall not hurt them, they shall lay hands upon the sick and they shall recover: and they went forth preaching everywhere, the Lord co-operating, and confirming the Word by signs following" (xvi. 17–20). It is a miraculous and not a saving faith which is there understood. The Jewish nation only believed in Jehovah on account of His miracles; for they were external men, and these are only moved to divine worship, by things external, such as miracles which strike their minds. A miraculous faith was also the first faith with those with whom the new church was to be established. It is also the first with all in the Christian world at this day, wherefore the miracles performed by the Lord were described, and also are preached. The first faith with all is an historical faith, which afterwards becomes saving when man by his life becomes spiritual.

It is first of all to be believed, that the Lord is the God of heaven and earth, and that He is Omnipotent, Omnipresent, Omniscient, Infinite, and One with the Father; these things are necessary to be known, and so far as they are only known, they are historical. Historical faith causes the Lord to be present, because it is an intuition of the Lord from the quality of His Divinity. That faith does not save, until man lives the life of faith, which is charity, for he then wills and does the things which he believes, and to will and to do is of the love, and love conjoins him whom faith causes to be present.

Again, in Matthew: "Jesus said, verily I say unto you, if ye have faith as a grain of mustard seed, ye shall say to this mountain, Remove hence to yonder place, and it shall be removed, and nothing shall be impossible to you" (xvii. 14–20). In Mark: "Have the faith of God; verily I say unto you that whosoever shall say to this mountain, be thou lifted up, and cast into the sea, and shall not doubt in his heart, but shall believe that those things which he saith shall come to pass, he shall have whatsoever he saith: wherefore I say unto you, all things whatsoever ye desire when ye pray, believe that ye receive them, and ye shall receive them" (xi. 22, 23, 24). In Matthew: "Jesus said unto the disciples, if ye have faith and doubt not, ye shall not only do that which is done to this fig-tree, but also if ye shall say to this mountain, be thou lifted up and cast into the sea, it shall be done; yea, all things whatsoever ye shall ask, believing in Me, ye shall receive" (xxi. 21, 22). In Luke: "If ye have faith as a grain of a mustard seed, and shall say to this sycamore tree, be thou rooted up and planted in the sea, it shall obey you" (xvii. 6).

By faith is here understood faith from the Lord, wherefore it is called the faith of God, and they who are in faith from the Lord ask for nothing but what conduces to the Lord's kingdom and their own salvation. Other things they do not desire, for they say in their hearts, why should we ask for anything that is not of such use? They cannot have the faith of God or faith from the Lord in asking anything but what it is given them from the Lord to ask. It is impossible for the angels of heaven to desire, and consequently to ask, anything else, and if they should, they could not possibly have any faith that they should receive it.

The Lord compared such faith to the ability and power of casting a mountain or a sycamore tree into the sea, because the Lord in this, as well as in other parts of the Word, spake by correspondences, wherefore those words are also to be understood spiritually. By a mountain is signified the love of self and of the world, thus the love of evil. By a sycamore tree is signified the faith of that love, which is a faith of the false from evil. By the sea is signified hell. By plucking up a mountain, and casting it into the sea by the faith of God, is signified to cast those loves, which in themselves are diabolical, into hell, and in like manner the faith of the false from evil, which is effected by faith from the Lord.

Passages from the evangelists concerning saving faith, which is faith of truth from the Lord:—In John: "As Moses lifted up the serpent in the wilderness, so also must the Son of Man be lifted up, that whosoever believeth in Him may not perish, but have eternal life.

For God so loved the world, that He gave His only begotten Son, that whosoever believeth in Him may not perish but have eternal life. He who believeth in Him, is not judged, but he who believeth not, is already judged, because he hath not believed in the name of the only begotten Son of God" (iii. 14–19). "The Father loveth the Son, and hath given all things into His hand; he who believeth in the Son hath eternal life, but he who believeth not in the Son shall not see life, but the anger of God abideth on him" (iii. 35, 36). "Unless ye believe that I am, ye shall die in your sins" (viii. 24). "They said unto Jesus, what shall we do that we may work the works of God? Jesus answering said, this is the work of God, that ye believe in Him whom the Father hath sent. I am the bread of life; he who cometh to Me shall not hunger, and he who believeth in Me shall never thirst. This is the will of Him who sent Me, that every one who seeth the Son, and believeth in Him, may have eternal life, and I will raise him up at the last day. No one hath seen the Father, except he Who is with the Father, He hath seen the father: verily I say unto you, he who believeth in Me hath eternal life: I am the bread of life") vi. 29, 33, 35, 36, 40, 47, 48). "Jesus said, he who heareth My Word and believeth Him who sent Me, hath eternal life, and shall not come into judgment, but shall pass from death into life; verily I say unto you, that the hour shall come, when the dead shall hear the voice of the Son of God, and they who hear shall live: even as the Father hath life in Himself, so hath He given to the Son to have life in Himself" (v. 24, 25, 26). "Jesus said, if any man thirst, let him come to Me and drink; whosoever believeth in Me, as the Scripture saith, out of His belly shall flow rivers of living water: these things said he of the spirit, which they who believe in Him should receive" (vii. 37, 38, 39). "Jesus said, I am the resurrection and the life, he who believeth in Me, although he were dead, he shall live; but whosoever liveth and believeth in Me, shall not die eternally" (xi. 25, 26, 27). "Jesus cried, and said, he who believeth in Me, believeth not in Me but in Him who sent Me; I am come a light into the world, that every one who believeth in Me may not abide in darkness: and if any one hear My words, and yet believe not, I do not judge him; he who despiseth Me, and doth not receive My words, hath one that judgeth him, the Word, which I have spoken, shall judge him at the last day" (xii. 44–48). "As long as ye have the light, believe in the light, that ye may be the sons of the light" (xii. 36). "Let not your heart be troubled, believe in God and believe in Me" (xiv. 1). "As many as received him, to them gave He power to become the sons of God, believing in His name" (i. 12). "Many believed in His name, when they saw His signs" (ii. 23). "These things are written that ye may believe that Jesus is the Christ, the Son of God, and that believing ye may have life in his name" (xx. 31). In Mark: "Jesus said unto His disciples, go ye into all the world and preach the gospel to every creature; he who shall believe and be baptized, shall be saved, but he who believeth not shall be condemned" (xvi. 15, 16).

By believing in the Lord is signified not only to adore and worship Him, but also to live from Him. . . . To believe in Him is to believe that he regenerates man, and gives eternal life to those who are regenerated by Him. The same as is signified by believing in His name. . . . The quality of the Lord is the all of faith and love, whereby He effects man's salvation, for this quality is the essence which proceeds from Him. When this quality is thought of by man, then the Lord becomes present with him, and when this quality is loved, the Lord is then conjoined to him; hence it is, that they who believe in His name have eternal life.—APOCALYPSE REVEALED, 815.

V

PARTICULAR CAUSES OF DISEASE

That straitness of spirit is a state near desperation, may be manifest from this consideration, that they who are in a state near desperation have an external anxiety, and in such case are actually in straitness of spirit. Straitness of spirit, in the external sense, is a compression of the breast, and thence as it were a difficulty of respiration. In the internal sense it is an anxiety by reason of the deprivation of the truth which is of faith, and of the good which is of charity, and thence a state near desperation. A state of compression as to respiration, and anxiety on account of the deprivation of the truth of faith and the good of charity, correspond to each other, as a natural effect in the body grounded in a spiritual cause in the mind.

That the deprivation of spiritual truth and good produces such anxiety, and consequently such straitness, cannot be believed by those who are not in faith and charity, for these imagine that to be tormented on such account is weakness and sickliness of mind. They do not suppose that there is anything real in faith and charity, thus neither in those things which relate to their souls and to heaven, but only in opulence and eminence. They think also, what are faith and charity? are they not mere sounds? yea, what is conscience? to be tormented on account of these things is to be tormented on account of such things as man sees inwardly in himself from a delirium of phantasy, and hence supposes to be something and yet they are not; but what are opulence and eminence? these things we see with the eyes, and are convinced that they are, by the pleasure which they excite, for the whole body is expanded, and is replenished with joy arising from them. Thus merely natural men think, and thus amongst themselves they speak.

The spiritual account faith and charity to be the primary life. When they imagine themselves to be deprived of the truths and goods of faith and charity, they are affected with anguish, as they who are in the anguish of death, for they see before them spiritual death, that is, damnation.—HEAVENLY ARCANA, 7217.

PAIN—GRIEF—ANXIETY—FEAR

The lust of the flesh is from the love of self and of the world. Pain signifies this lust. Whilst man is purifying from those loves, as is the case whilst he is regenerating, he is in pain and anxiety; the lusts, which are at that time wiping away, being what grieve and suffer torment.

They, who are in no capacity of being reformed, are altogether ignorant of what it is to grieve on account of being deprived of truths, and suppose it impossible for any one to be troubled and tormented on such account. The sole cause of anxiety, in their imagination, is the loss of corporeal and worldly goods, as health, honour, fame, wealth, and life. They, who are in a capacity of being reformed, entertain other and contrary thoughts. They are preserved by the Lord in the affection of what is good, and in the thought of what is true, and therefore they come into anxiety when they are deprived of such affection and thought. It is well known, that all anxiety and grief arise solely from the deprivation of those things with which any one is affected, or which he loves. They who are affected only with corporeal and worldly things, or who love only such things, are made sensible of grief when they are deprived of them; but they who are affected with spiritual goods and truths, and who love these things, are made sensible of grief when they are deprived thereof, the life of every one being nothing but affection and love.—HEAVENLY ARCANA, 4496, 2689.

"Why are thou cast down, O my soul? and why art

thou disquieted within me? hope thou in God; for I
shall yet praise him, who is the health of my countenance, and my God" (Psalm xlii. 11; xliii. 5). The expression, "the health of my countenance," signifies all
things within, that is to say, all things of the mind and
affections, consequently, all things pertaining to love
and faith, which, because of their saving nature, are here
called health, the health of the countenance. The evil
affections, which are lusts, are also expressed in the Word
in the same manner, because they appear in the face,
for the face is the external or natural form of the interiors
of the soul and spirit. In the spiritual world they form
a one, for there it is not permitted to feign in the face
what does not really exist in the affections and thus in
the interiors of the mind. The angels of heaven have a
certain lustre and comeliness in the face, whereas with
the infernal spirits the face is dark and deformed.—APOCA-
LYPSE EXPLAINED, 412.

"Our God shall come, and shall not keep silence; a
fire shall devour before him, and it shall be very tempes-
tuous round about him" (Psalm l. 3). And in Hosea:
"For they have sown the wind, and they shall reap the
whirlwind" (viii. 7). In these passages by storms and
tempests is signified the dispersion of falsities and evils,
because they who are principled in the falsities of evil
are cast down into hell by a stormy wind. Again, in
David: "They that go down into the sea in ships, that
do business in great waters; these see the works of Jehovah, and his wonders in the deep. For he command-
eth, and raiseth the stormy wind, which lifteth up the
waves thereof. He maketh the storm a calm, so that
the waves thereof are still" (Psalm cvii. 23, 24, 25, 29).

These things are said concerning temptations and lib-
erations from them; by the stormy wind, and the waves
of the sea being thereby lifted up, are signified temptations, inasmuch as spiritual temptations are occasioned
by the irruption of falsities into the thoughts, whence
arise remorse of conscience and grief of mind, which are

signified by the stormy wind rising and lifting up the waves; liberation from them is signified by, "He maketh the storm a calm, so that the waves thereof are still." The same is signified by these words in Mark: "And there arose a great storm of wind, and the waves beat into the ship, so that it was now full. And he was in the hinder part of the ship, asleep on a pillow; and they awake him, and say unto him, Master, carest thou not that we perish? And he arose, and rebuked the wind, and said unto the sea, Peace, be still. And the wind ceased, and there was a great calm" (iv. 37, 38, 39). Also in Luke: "But as they sailed he fell asleep; and there came down a storm of wind on the lake, and they were filled with water, and were in jeopardy. And they came to him, and awoke him, saying Master, master, we perish. Then he arose, and rebuked the wind and the raging of the water: and they ceased, and there was a calm" (viii. 23, 24).

The miracle here adduced involves the temptations of the spiritual man: the great storm of wind that arose causing the waves to beat into the ship, so that it was full, signifies those temptations: deliverance from them is signified by Jesus being awakened when they were in extreme fear; and by his rebuking the wind, and saying to the sea, "Peace, be still," and there was a great calm. Every word also contains a spiritual sense: the great storm of wind here mentioned signifies temptations, which are irruptions of falsities, or inundations of the mind by falsities. This is also evident from the rebuke of the wind and the waves, and from the words of the Lord to the sea, "Peace, be still," as being said to those things, or to those who induce temptations.

The winds which exist in the spiritual world, appear to arise there from different quarters, some from the south, some from the north, and some from the east; those which are from the south disperse truths with those who are in falsities, and those which are from the east disperse goods with those who are in evils. The reason

of the winds dispersing them is, because winds exist from
a strong and powerful influx of the divine principle
through the heavens into the lower parts of the spiritual
world, and where the influx comes, it fills truths and
goods, that is, it fills those who are in truths and goods
with the Divine principle as to their soul and spirit.
Those whose interiors consist merely of falsities and evils,
and their exteriors, of truths mixed with falsities and
goods mixed with evils, cannot sustain such influx from
the Divine principle. They betake themselves to their
own falsities and evils which they love, and reject the
truths and goods which they do not love, except for the
sake of self and of appearance.—APOCALYPSE EXPLAINED,
419.

"And God shall wipe away all tears from their eyes."
Hereby is signified a state of beatitude from the affection
of truth after falsities are removed by temptations. All
the beatitude which the angels enjoy is by truth from
good. The reason why all the beatitude of angels is
from this origin is, because divine truth proceeding from
the Lord is what constitutes heaven in general and in
particular, wherefore they who are in divine truths are
in the life of heaven, consequently in eternal beatitude.
Tears from the eyes signify grief of mind on account of
falsities and from falsities because by the eye is signified
the understanding of truth; and hence tears from the
eyes signify grief on account of there being no understanding of truth, consequently, on account of falsities.

Weeping is grief of heart. It bursts forth from the
heart, and breaks out into lamentations through the
mouth. Shedding of tears is grief of mind. It issues
forth from the thought through the eyes. In the act
both of weeping and of shedding tears water comes forth,
but bitter and astringent, and this is occasioned by the
influx from the spiritual world into the grief of man,
where bitter water corresponds to the defect of truth
because of falsities, and to grief on account thereof.—
APOCALYPSE EXPLAINED, 484.

All joy and all gladness is of love; for every one rejoices and is glad when his love is favoured, and when he arrives at and obtains the object of his love; in a word, all the joy of man proceeds from his love, and all sadness and grief of mind from opposition thereto.— APOCALYPSE EXPLAINED, 660.

With those who are about to be regenerated, the case is this: first of all they are in a state of tranquillity, or external peace. It is produced from a Divine state of peace, which is intimately within it, and exists in externals by the removal of lusts and falsities, for these are what cause all restlessness. Every man is in a state of tranquillity in the beginning of his life or in infancy, but in proportion as he advances in life, or grows up to manhood, in the same proportion he removes himself from that state, because he gives himself up to worldly cares, and thence to anxieties, by the lusts of self-love and the love of the world, and by the falsities therein originating. Nearly similar to this is the new life of a regenerate man. In the beginning he is in a state of tranquillity, but as he passes into a new life, he also passes at the same time into an untranquil state. The evil and false principles, which he had before imbibed, emerge and come forth, and disturb him, and this to such a degree at length, that he is immersed in temptations and vexations arising from the diabolical crew, who are continually striving to destroy the state of his new life. Nevertheless in the inmost ground of his spirit he is in a state of peace, for unless he was in such a state in his inmost principles, he would not engage in combat, inasmuch as he has continual respect to that state, as an end, in the combats wherein he is engaged, and unless he had such an end, he would in no wise have power and strength to engage in combat; hence also it is that he overcomes. Inasmuch as this state of peace is the end regarded, he also comes into this state after combats or temptations.— HEAVENLY ARCANA, 3696.

Fear is in general two-fold, fear in a principle not holy

and fear in an holy principle. This latter fear is called holy fear, being grounded in admiration respecting what is divine, and also in love. Love without holy fear is like somewhat unsavoury, or like meat unseasoned with salt, and consequently insipid; but love with fear is like salted meat which yet does not taste of salt. The fear of love is, lest in any manner the Lord should suffer hurt, or a neighbour; thus lest in any manner good and truth should suffer hurt, consequently the holy principle of love and faith, and thence of worship.

According to the proportion of good and truth in which any one is principled, the same is the proportion of his fear lest good and truth should suffer hurt, nevertheless in the same proportion it does not appear as fear. In proportion as the love of good and truth is small in any one, in the same proportion he has less of fear concerning good and truth, and in the same proportion it appears not as love, but as fear, and hence such have fear respecting hell. But where there is nothing of the love of good and truth, there is nothing of holy fear, but only fear for the loss of honour, of gain, of reputation on account of good and truth, also of punishments and death, which fear is external, and especially affects the body and natural man, and the thoughts thereof; whereas the former fear, namely, holy fear, especially affects the spirit or internal man, and the conscience thereof.—HEAVENLY ARCANA, 3718.

VI

SPIRITUAL POWER

Those who think of angelic power, especially of the power of the archangels mentioned in the Word, from natural light not illuminated by the light of heaven, because without a medium, and particularly if there be not correspondence, cannot form any other idea of it, than as of the power of the mighty in the world, viz., that they have many thousands of inferiors over whom they bear rule, and that eminent stations in heaven consist in such rule. Angelic power indeed exceeds all the power of the mighty in the world, and it is so great, that one of the inferior angels can drive away myriads of infernals, and thrust them down into their hells, hence also in the Word they are called powers and also dominions. The least of them is the greatest; He is most powerful, who believes, wills, and perceives that all power is from the Lord, and none from himself.—HEAVENLY ARCANA, 5428.

All ability, such as the power of thinking and willing, of perceiving, of doing good, of believing, of dissipating falses and evils, is from good through truth; good is the principal, and truth is only the instrumental.—HEAVENLY ARCANA, 6343.

All ability in the spiritual world is from good by truth; without good, truth has no ability at all, for truth is as the body, and good is as the soul of that body, and the soul, to effect anything, must act through the body: hence it is evident, that truth without good has no ability at all, as the body without the soul has no ability, for the body in such case is a carcass; so also is truth without good.

Scarcely any one in the world can know what is meant by ability belonging to truth from good, but it is known to those who are in the other life, thus by revelation

thence. They are in faith from charity, are in ability
by truth from good; in this ability are all the angels.
In the Word angels are called abilities, or powers, for
they are in the ability of restraining evil spirits, even
one angel a thousand together; they exercise their
ability chiefly with man, by defending him occasionally
against several hells, and this by a thousand and a thousand methods. This ability they have by the truth
of faith derived from the good of charity; but as they
have faith from the Lord, the Lord alone is the ability
in them.—HEAVENLY ARCANA, 6344.

They who are principled in doctrinals and not so much
in life, know no other than that the kingdom of heaven
is similar to kingdoms on earth in this respect, that authority over others therein constitutes greatness, the
delight arising from such authority being the only delight
with which they are acquainted, wherefore the Lord
spake also according to this appearance, as in Matthew,
"Whosoever doeth and teacheth, he shall be called great
in the kingdom of the heavens," v. 19; and in David,
"I have said, Ye are gods, and ye are all the sons of the
Highest," lxxxii. 6; John x. 34, 35. Inasmuch as the
disciples themselves had at first no other sentiments
respecting the kingdom of heaven, than such as were
grounded in earthly greatness and pre-eminence, as appears from Matt. chap. xviii. 1; Mark ix. 34; Luke ix.
46; and also had an idea of sitting on the right-hand and
the left of a king, Matt. xx. 20, 21, 24; Mark x. 37;
therefore also the Lord replied according to their appre-
hension and idea, saying (when they disputed which of
them should be greatest), "Ye shall eat and drink on
My table in My kingdom, and shall sit on thrones, judging
the twelve tribes of Israel," Luke xxii. 24, 30; Matt.
xix. 28. At this time they did not know that heavenly
delight was not a delight grounded in greatness and pre-
eminence, but a delight grounded in humiliation and the
affection of serving others, consequently in a desire of
being the least and not the greatest.

They who are principled in the science of knowledges, and not in the life of charity, cannot know that there exists any delight but what results from pre-eminence. Inasmuch as this is the only delight of which they have any idea, they are altogether ignorant of heavenly delight resulting from humiliation and an affection of being serviceable to others. In heaven all become great, pre-eminent, powerful, and of authority, for one angel has greater power than myriads of infernal spirits, yet not of himself, but from the Lord: and only so far from the Lord, as he believes that he has no power self-derived, and thus that he is least; and this he may believe, so far as he is in humiliation, and the affection of being serviceable.—HEAVENLY ARCANA, 3417.

They who are in things external separate from what is internal, have nothing of power to resist the evils and falses which are from hell, because all power of resisting those things is from the Divine.—HEAVENLY ARCANA, 10481.

That all the power of truth is from the good of love cannot be apprehended by those who have only a material idea concerning power. In the heavens all power is derived from Divine Truth proceeding from the Divine Good of the Lord, hence the angels have power, for the angels are receptions of Divine Truth from the Lord. By power they protect man, removing the hells from him, for one angel prevails against a thousand who are from the hells. . . . That truths derived from good have all power, and *vice versa*, that falses derived from evil have no power, is a thing most known in the other life. That truths derived from good have such power, cannot be apprehended by those who have an idea of truth and of its faith as of a principle of thought alone, when yet man's principle of thought derived from his will principle makes all the strength of his body.—HEAVENLY ARCANA, 10482.

VII

POWERLESSNESS OF EVIL

What is in good and at the same time in truth is
something; and what is evil and at the same time
false is not any thing. By its not being any thing
is meant that it has no power and no spiritual life. Those
who are in evil and at the same time in falsity, have
indeed power with one another; for one who is evil can
do evil, and he also does it in a thousand ways; nevertheless, he can do evil to the evil only from [their] evil;
but he cannot do the least evil to the good, except, as
is sometimes the case, by conjunction with their evil.
From this come temptations, which are infestations by
the evil who are with one, and the combats thence arising, whereby the good can be freed from their evils.
Since the evil have no power, all hell before the Lord is
not only as nothing, but is absolutely nothing in power.

It is wonderful that the wicked all believe themselves to be powerful, and the good all believe themselves
to be without power. This is because the evil attribute
all things to their own power, and thus to cunning and
malice, and attribute nothing to the Lord. The good
attribute nothing to their own prudence, but all to the
Lord who is Almighty. Furthermore, evil and falsity
together are not anything, because there is no spiritual
life in them; for this reason the life of the infernals is
not called life, but death; therefore, since every real
thing is of life, there cannot be any real thing which is
of death.—DIVINE PROVIDENCE, 19.

It is said in John, In the beginning was the Word and
the Word was with God, and God was the Word. . . . All
things were made through Him, and without Him was
not any thing made that was made. In Him was life,

and the life was the light of men. ... He was in the world and the world was made through Him. ... And the Word was made flesh and dwelt among us, and we beheld His glory (i. 1–14). That it is the Lord who is meant by the Word is plain, for it is said that the Word was made flesh; but what is more particularly meant by the Word has not yet been known, and so is to be told. The Word in this passage is the Divine truth, which is in the Lord and from the Lord. For this reason He is also called the light, which is the Divine truth. In heaven the Divine truth has all power, and without it there is no power at all. All angels from the Divine truth are called powers, and are powers just so far as they are recipients or receptacles of it. By it they prevail over the hells and over all who oppose them. A thousand enemies there cannot stand against a single ray of the light of heaven, which is Divine truth. And because angels are angels from their reception of Divine truth, it follows that the whole heaven is from no other source, since heaven consists of angels. That there is so great power in Divine truth those cannot believe who have no other idea of truth than as of thought or speech, in which there is no power in itself, except as others do it from obedience. But in Divine truth there is power in itself, and such power that by means of it heaven is created and the world is created, with all things therein.

That there is such power in Divine truth may be illustrated by the power of truth and good in man, and by the power of light and heat from the sun in the world. All things that man does, he does from his understanding and will, from the will by means of good and from the understanding by means of truth. From good and truth, man moves his whole body, and a thousand things therein rush with one accord to do their will and pleasure. The whole body is formed for subservience to and is formed from good and truth. By the power of heat and light from the sun in the world—since all things that grow in the world, as trees, grain, flowers, grasses, fruits, and seeds, exist in no other way than by the heat and light of the sun; from which it is manifest what power of production there is in that heat and light.

What then must be the power in Divine light, which is Divine truth, and in Divine heat, which is Divine good! from which because heaven exists, the world also exists. From these things it may be evident how it is to be understood that all things were made through the Word, that is, through the Divine truth from the Lord. For the same reason in the book of creation, light is first spoken of and then the things that are from the light (Gen. i. 3, 4). Hence also all things in the universe both in heaven and in the world, have reference to good and truth and to their conjunction, in order to be any thing.—HEAVEN AND HELL, 137-138.

That angels have power those cannot understand who know nothing of the spiritual world, and of its influx into the natural world. They think that angels cannot have power because they are spiritual, and so pure and unsubstantial that they cannot even be seen with the eyes. But those who look more interiorly into the causes of things, take a different view. They know that all the power which man has, is from his understanding and will—for without these he cannot move a particle of his body—and the understanding and will are his spiritual man. This moves the body and its members at its pleasure; for what it thinks, that the mouth and tongue speak, and what it wills, this the body does; it also gives strength at pleasure. The will and understanding of man are ruled by the Lord through angels and spirits, and therefore all things of the body also are so ruled, because they are from the will and understanding; and man cannot even stir a step without the influx of heaven. Every man is so ruled, and he may know this from the doctrine of the Church and from the Word, for he prays that God may send His angels to lead him, direct his steps, teach him, and inspire what he should think and what he should speak; though when he thinks by himself without doctrine, he says and believes otherwise.

But in the spiritual world the power of angels is so great, that if I should bring forward all that I have seen in regard to it, it would exceed belief. If anything there resists, which is to be removed because contrary to Divine order, they cast it down and overturn it merely by an effort of the will and a look. I have seen also some hundreds of thousands of evil spirits dispersed by them and cast into hell. Numbers are of no avail against them, nor arts, cunning, and leagues, for they see all, and disperse them in a moment. Such power have angels in the spiritual world. That they have similar power in the natural world too, when it is granted, is evident from the Word—as that they gave whole armies to destruction, and that they brought a pestilence of which seventy thousand men died. Of this angel we read: The angel stretched out his hand against Jerusalem to destroy it; but Jehovah repented Him of the evil, and said to the angel that destroyed the people, It is enough, stay now thy hand. And David saw the angel that smote the people (2 Sam. xxiv. 16, 17).

It is to be known, however, that angels have no power at all from themselves, but that all their power is from the Lord; and that they are only so far powers as they acknowledge this. Whoever of them believes that he has power from himself, becomes instantly so weak that he cannot even resist one evil spirit; which is the cause that angels attribute nothing at all of merit to themselves, that they are averse to all praise and glory on account of anything done, and that they ascribe the praise and glory to the Lord.

It is Divine truth proceeding from the Lord which has all power in the heavens, for the Lord in heaven is Divine truth, united to Divine good. As far as angels are receptions of this truth, so far they are powers. Every one also is his own truth and his own good, because every one is such as his understanding and will are.—HEAVEN AND HELL, 228-231.

VIII

HEALING AND MIRACLES

Divine miracles differ from magical miracles, as heaven
from hell; divine miracles proceed from divine truth,
and go forward according to order, the effects in ultimates are miracles when it pleases the Lord that they
should be presented in that form. All divine miracles
represent states of the Lord's kingdom in the heavens,
and of the Lord's kingdom in the earths, or of the church;
this is the internal form of divine miracles; so is the case
with all the miracles in Egypt, and also with the rest that
are mentioned in the Word. The miracles which the
Lord himself wrought when he was in the world, signified
the approaching state of the church; as the opening the
eyes of the blind, the ears of the deaf, the tongues of the
dumb, the lame walking, the maimed and also the lepers
being healed, signified that such as are represented by
the blind, the deaf, the dumb, the lame, the maimed, the
leprous, would receive the gospel, and be spiritually
healed, and this by the coming of the Lord into the world.

Magical miracles involve nothing at all, being wrought
by the evil to acquire to themselves power over others.
They appear in the external form like to divine miracles;
the reason is, because they flow from order, and order appears like in the ultimates where miracles are presented.
For example, the divine truth proceeding from the Lord
has in it all power, hence it is, that there is also power
in truths in the ultimates of order; therefore the evil
acquire to themselves power by truths, and gain dominion
over others. Take another example; it is according to
order, that states of affection and thought cause the idea
of place and distance in the other life, and that the in-
habitants appear to be so far distant from each other,
as they are in a diverse state; this law, or principle of

order, is from the Divine Being, that all who are in the
Grand Man may be distinct from each other; magicians in
the other life abuse this law or principle of order, for
they induce in others changes of state, and thereby trans-
late them at one time aloft, at another time into the deep,
and also cast them together into societies, that they may
serve them for subjects. Magical miracles, although in
the external form they appear like unto divine miracles,
nevertheless have inwardly in them a contrary end, viz.,
of destroying those things which are of the church,
whereas divine miracles have inwardly in them the end
of building up those things which are of the church.—
HEAVENLY ARCANA, 7337.

"Jesus said unto the disciples, these signs shall follow
them that believe; in my name they shall cast out
demons; they shall speak with new tongues; they shall
take up serpents; if they drink any deadly thing, it shall
not hurt them; they shall lay hands on the infirm, and
they shall recover. And they went out and preached
everywhere, the Lord working with them by signs following" (Mark xvi. 17, 18, 20). Although these were
miracles, yet they were called signs, because they testified
of the divine power of the Lord who operated them,
wherefore it is said, the Lord working with them by those
signs. They would have been called miracles, if applied
to the evil, for with them such things only induce a stupor
and strike the mind, and yet do not persuade to believe.
The case is otherwise with the good, for with these the
same things are testifications which persuade to believe,
wherefore also they are called signs, and it is said, these
signs shall follow them that believe.

Those miraculous signs, as that they should cast out
demons, speak with new tongues, take up serpents, that
if they drank any deadly thing it should not hurt them,
and that they should restore the sick by the laying on of
hands, were in their essence and in their origin spiritual,
from which those things flowed and came forth as effects:
for they were correspondences, which derive their all

from the spiritual world by influx from the Lord. That
they should cast out demons in the name of the Lord,
derived all its effects from this circumstance, that the
name of the Lord spiritually understood is the all of
doctrine out of the Word from the Lord, and that demons
are falses of every kind, which are so cast out, that is,
removed, by doctrine out of the Word from the Lord;
that they should speak with new tongues, derives its
effect from this, that new tongues denote doctrinals for
the new church; that they should take up serpents was,
because serpents signify the hells as to malice, and so
that they should be safe from the infestation thereof;
that they should not be hurt if they drank the deadly
thing, denoted that the malice of the hells should not in-
fect them; and their restoring the infirm by laying on of
hands, signified, that by communication and conjunction
with heaven, thus with the Lord, they should restore
to health from spiritual diseases, which are called iniquities and sins, the laying on of the hands of the disciples
corresponding to communication and conjunction with
the Lord, and so as to the removal of iniquities by His
divine power.—APOCALYPSE EXPLAINED, 706.

By the dumb whom the Lord healed are signified the
nations, which by his coming into the world were delivered from falses and consequent evils; as by the dumb
in Matthew, "Lo, they brought to him a man that was
dumb, obsessed by a demon, but when the demon was
cast out the dumb spake," ix. 32, 33; and again, "There
was brought to Jesus one obsessed by a demon, blind and
dumb, and he healed him, so that the blind and dumb
both spake and saw," xii. 22; in like manner by the dumb
also obsessed by a demon, in Mark ix. 17 to 30. It is
to be noted, that the miracles wrought by the Lord all
signify the state of the church, and of the human race
saved by his coming into the world, viz., that on this
occasion they were delivered from hell who received the
faith of charity; these things are involved in the Lord's
miracles: in general, all the miracles which are recorded

in the Old Testament signify the state of the Lord's church and kingdom; in this divine miracles are distinguished from diabolical or magical miracles, howsoever they appear alike in the external form, as was the case with the miracles of the magicians in Egypt.— APOCALYPSE EXPLAINED, 6988.

Hearing corresponds both to perception and obedience: to perception, because the things which are heard are inwardly perceived, and to obedience, because it is hence known what ought to be done. In the Word, by the deaf are also signified the nations which do not know the truth of faith, because they have not the Word, and therefore they cannot live according to those truths, nevertheless when they are instructed, they receive them, and live according to them; these are meant in Isaiah, "Then shall be opened the eyes of the blind, and the ears of the deaf shall be opened," xxxv. 5. Again, "Hear, ye deaf, and ye blind look in seeing," xlii. 18, 19, 20. Again, "In that day the deaf shall hear the words of the book, and out of thick darkness, and out of darkness shall the eyes of the blind see," xxix. 18. Again, "Bring forth the blind people who have eyes, and the deaf who have ears," xliii. 8, 9: by the deaf in these passages are meant those who by the Lord's coming came into a state of receiving the truths of faith, that is, of perceiving them and obeying them. The same are signified by the deaf whom the Lord healed, see Mark vii. 31; ix. 25. In consequence of this signification of the deaf, it was forbidden those, amongst whom the representative church was instituted, to curse the deaf, and put a stumbling block before the blind, Levit. xix. 14.—APOCALYPSE EXPLAINED, 6989.

By the blind in the Word are also signified the nations which live in ignorance of the truth which is of faith, because out of the church, but who when instructed receive faith; the same are also signified by the blind whom the Lord healed, see Matt. ix. 27 to 31; xii. 22; xx. 29 to the end; xxi. 14; Mark viii. 22 to 37; x. 46 to the end; Luke xviii. 35 to the end; John ix. 1 to the end.

That such things as are signified by the dumb, by the deaf, and by the blind, also by the mouth and by the seeing, exist with man by virtue of an influx of life from Jehovah or the Lord; for hence exist both evils and goods with every one, but evils from man and goods from the Lord. The reason why evils exist from man, is, because the life which flows-in from the Lord, that is, good and truth, is turned by man into evil and the false, thus into what is contrary to life, which is called spiritual death. It appears as if the Lord also induces evil, because he gives life, therefore from the appearance evil is attributed in the Word to Jehovah or the Lord.—APOCALYPSE EXPLAINED, 6990

The Lord, when He was in the world, and united His Human to the Divine itself, abrogated the sabbath as to representative worship, or as to the worship which prevailed amongst the Israelitish people, and made the sabbath day a day of instruction in the doctrine of faith and love. This is involved in what is written in John, "Jesus healing a certain person on the sabbath day, said to him, take up thy bed and walk; and he took up his bed and walked." The Jews said, that it was not allowed to carry a bed on the sabbath day, and they sought to kill the Lord, because He broke the sabbath, v. 8, 9, 10, 11, 18. By healing a sick person is signified the purification of man from evils and the falses of evil; by a bed is signified doctrine; and by walking is signified life. That all the healings of diseases, which were performed by the Lord, involve purifications from evils and falses, or restorations of spiritual life.—HEAVENLY ARCANA, 10362.

By the Lord saying to those sick men, Arise, take up thy bed, and walk, is signified doctrine, and a life according thereto. The bed signifies doctrine, and to walk signifies life. A sick person signifies those who have transgressed and sinned; wherefore the Lord said to the sick man at the pool of Bethesda, Behold, thou art made whole; sin no more, lest a worse thing come unto thee; and to the paralytic let down in a bed through the roof, Whether is it easier to say, thy sins are forgiven thee, or to say, Arise, take up thy bed, and walk. They who do not understand the internal sense of the Word, may suppose that the words which the Lord spake involve nothing more than what appears in the sense of the letter, when, nevertheless, the whole contains in it a spiritual sense, for he spake from the divine principle, and thus before heaven at the same time as before the world.—APOCALYPSE EXPLAINED, 163.

IX

INFLUX

CONJUNCTION OF HEAVEN WITH MAN

That man is governed by the Lord through spirits is because he is not in the order of heaven, for he is born into the opposite of Divine order. He is therefore to be reduced into order, and he cannot be so reduced except mediately through spirits. It would be otherwise if man were born into the good which is according to the order of heaven; then he would be governed by means of order itself, thus by the general influx. By means of this influx man is governed as to the things which proceed from thought and will into act, thus as to speech and as to actions; for these flow according to natural order, with which therefore the spirits who are adjoined to man have nothing in common. By means of the general influx from the spiritual world animals also are governed, because they are in the order of their life; nor have they been able to pervert and destroy it, because they have no rational faculty.

As to what further concerns the conjunction of heaven with the human race, it is to be known that the Lord Himself flows in with every man, according to the order of heaven, both into his inmosts and into his outmosts, or ultimates, and disposes him for receiving heaven, and governs his ultimates from his inmosts, and at the same time the inmosts from his ultimates, and thus holds all things with him in connection. This influx of the Lord is called immediate influx, but the other influx, which takes place through spirits, is called mediate influx; the latter subsists by means of the former. Immediate influx, which is of the Lord Himself, is from His Divine Human, and is into man's will, and through his will into his understanding, or what is the same thing, into his love, and through the love into his faith. This Divine influx is perpetual, and is received in good with the good, but not with the evil. With the evil it is either rejected, or suffocated, or perverted; hence they have an evil life, which in the spiritual sense is death.

The spirits who are with man, as well those who are conjoined to heaven as those who are conjoined to hell, never flow in from their own memory and its thought with man; for if they should flow in from their own thought, man would not know otherwise than that the things which are theirs were his own. But still through them there flows in with man from heaven, affection which is of love for what is good and true, and from hell, affection which is of love for what is evil and false. As far therefore as man's affection agrees with what flows in, so far it is received by him in his own thought, for man's interior though is altogether according to his affection or love; but as far as it does not agree, so far it is not received. Since thought does not flow into man through spirits, but only affection for good and affection for evil, man has choice, because he has freedom; thus that he can with thought receive good and reject evil, for he knows from the Word what is good and what is evil. What he receives with thought from affection, is also appropriated to him; but what he does not receive with thought from affection, is not appropriated to him.

It has also been given to know whence man has anxiety, grief of mind, and interior sadness which is called melancholy. There are spirits who are not as yet in conjunction with hell, because still in their first state. These spirits love things undigested and corrupt, as of putrefying food in the stomach. They are present with such things in man, because they find enjoyment in them, and they talk there with one another from their own evil affection. The affection of their speech flows

in from this source into man, which affection, if it be
contrary to the man's own, becomes in him sadness
and melancholy anxiety; but if it be agreeable, it becomes in him gladness and cheerfulness. That anxiety of mind is thus produced, has been given me to
know and to be assured from much experience. I
have seen them, I have heard them, I have felt the
anxieties arising from them, I have spoken with them;
they have been driven away, and the anxiety ceased;
they have returned, and the anxiety returned; and I
have percived the increase and decrease of it, according
to their approach and removal. From this it has been
evident to me why it is that some who do not know
what conscience is, because they have no conscience,
ascribe its pangs to the stomach.

The conjunction of heaven with man is not as the
conjunction of man with man, but is a conjunction with
the interiors of his mind, thus with his spiritual or internal man. With his natural or external man there
is a conjunction by correspondences.

The man of the Church indeed says that all good is
from God, and that angels are with man; but yet few
believe that angels are conjoined to man, still less that
they are in his thought and affection. The word teaches
of heaven and its conjunction with man. There is
such conjunction that man cannot think the least thing
without spirits adjoined to him, and his spiritual life
depends on it. The cause of the ignorance on this
subject is that man believes he lives from himself, without connection with the First Esse of life, and does not
know that this connection is by means of the heavens.
If man believed, as is really the case, that all good is
from the Lord and all evil from hell, then he would not
make the good in him a matter of merit, neither would
evil be imputed to him; for thus in all the good which
he thinks and does he would look to the Lord, and all
the evil which flows in would be rejected to hell, whence
it comes. But because man does not believe this, and

thus supposes that all things which he thinks and wills are in himself and from himself, he appropriates evil to himself, and the good which flows in he defiles with merit.—HEAVEN AND HELL, 296–302.

CONJUNCTION OF HEAVEN WITH MAN BY THE WORD

Those who think from interior reason can see that there is a connection of all things by intermediates with the First, and that whatever is not in connection is dissipated. For they know when they think, that nothing can subsist from itself, but from what is prior to itself, thus all things from the First; and that the connection with what is prior is as the connection of an effect with its efficient cause; for when the efficient cause is taken away from its effect, then the effect is dissolved and destroyed. Because the learned thought thus, they saw and said that subsistence is perpetual existence; thus that all things subsist from the First, from Which because they have had their existence, they perpetually exist—that is, subsist. But what is the connection of everything with that which is prior to itself, thus with the First, from Which are all things, cannot be told in a few words, because it is various and diverse; it can only be told in general that there is a connection of the natural world with the spiritual world, and that in consequence there is a correspondence of all things in the natural world with all things in the spiritual; also that there is a connection and thence a correspondence of all things of man with all things of heaven.

Man is so created that he has connection and conjunction with the Lord, but only fellowship with the angels of heaven; that he has only fellowship, is because man from creation is like an angel as to the interiors of the mind. Hence it is that a man after death, if he has lived according to Divine order, becomes an angel, and then has the wisdom of angels. When therefore the conjunction of man with heaven is spoken of, his conjunction with the Lord and fellowship with angels is meant; for heaven is not heaven from what is the angels' own, but from the Lord's Divine.

The Divine influx of the Lord does not stop in the middle but proceeds to its ultimates. Since the middle through which it passes is the angelic heaven, and the ultimate is with man, and since there is nothing given which is unconnected, it follows that such is the connection and conjunction of heaven with the human race that the one subsists from the other, and that it would be with the human race without heaven as with a chain when the hook is removed, and with heaven without the human race as with a house without a foundation.

But because man has broken this connection with heaven by turning his interiors away from heaven and turning them to the world and himself, through love of self and the world, and thus withdrawing himself so as no longer to serve heaven for a basis and foundation, a medium has been provided by the Lord to be to heaven in the place of a basis and foundation, and also for the conjunction of heaven with man. This medium is the Word.—HEAVEN AND HELL, 303–305.

INFLUX AND DISEASE

All influx from the spiritual world varies according to reception, or according to the forms into which it flows, just as does the heat and light from the sun of the world. When the heat or love from it flows into good, as with good men and spirits and angels, it makes their good fruitful; but when it flows in with the wicked, it produces a contrary effect, for their evils either suffocate it or pervert it. In like manner the light of heaven when it flows into the truths of good, gives intelligence and wisdom; but when it flows into the falsities of evil, it is there turned into insanities and phantasies of various kinds—in all cases according to reception.—HEAVEN AND HELL, 569.

X

PROVIDENTIAL USE OF DISEASE

In the representative Church it was a common cere-
mony to wash the feet with water, thereby to signify,
that the filth of the natural man should be washed away.
The filth of the natural man are all those things which
relate to self-love and the love of the world. When
this filth is washed away, then goodnesses and truths
flow-in, for this filth is what alone prevents the influx
of good and of truth from the Lord. Good is continually flowing-in from the Lord, but when it comes through
the internal or spiritual man to his external or natural
man, it is there either perverted, or reflected back, or
suffocated. When the things appertaining to self-love
and the love of the world are removed, then good is there
received, and there fructifies, for then man exercises
himself in works of charity. This may appear from
many considerations, as from the state of man in mis-
fortune, misery, and disease, when the things appertaining to the external or natural man are laid asleep,
in which case man begins instantly to think piously,
and to will what is good, and also to exercise himself
in works of piety to the utmost of his ability; but when
the state is changed, there is a change also in these
things.—HEAVENLY ARCANA, 3147.

Manasseh in the original tongue signifies forgetfulness,
thus in the internal sense removal, viz., of evils as well
actual as hereditary, for when these are removed there
arises a new will-principle. The new will-principle exists by the influx of good from the Lord, which influx
is continual with man, but evils as well actual as hereditary are what hinder and oppose its reception. That
the new will-principle exists in such cases, appears manifest with those who are in misfortunes, miseries, and

diseases. On these occasions there is a removal of self-love and the love of the world, from which all evils flow, therefore a man at such times thinks well of God and his neighbour, and also is well disposed towards the latter; in like manner in temptations, which are spiritual griefs, and consequent interior miseries and despair; by these more especially the removal of evils is effected, and after evils are removed, celestial good from the Lord flows-in, whence comes the new will-principle in the natural, which in the representative sense is Manasseh.—HEAVENLY ARCANA, 5353.

XI

DIVINE ORDER

God himself cannot do contrary to his own divine order,
since this would be to do contrary to Himself. Wherefore he leads every man according to Himself, or according
to order, and the wandering and backsliding into it,
and the disobedient to it. If man could have been
created without free agency in spiritual things, what
then would be easier for Almighty God, than to bring
all in the whole world to believe in the Lord? Could
He not have brought this faith into every one, both
immediately and mediately; immediately by his absolute power, and its irresistible operation, which is continual, that man may be saved; or mediately, by tor-
ments injected into his conscience, by mortal convulsions
of the body, and grievous threats of death, if he did not
receive it; and besides, by opening hell, and thence by
the presence of devils holding in their hands terrible
torches; or by calling out thence the dead whom they
had known, under the image of frightful spectres? But
to these things it is answered from the words of Abraham
to the rich man in hell; If they hear not Moses and the
prophets, neither will they be persuaded if one should
rise from the dead, Luke xvi. 31.

It is asked at this day, why miracles are not done,
as formerly; for it is believed that if they were done,
every one would, in heart, acknowledge. But the reason that miracles are not done at this day, as before,
is because miracles force, and take away free agency in
spiritual things, and from spiritual make man natural.
Every one in the Christian world, since the coming of
the Lord, may become spiritual, and he is made spiritual
solely by Him through the Word; but the faculty for
this would be lost, if man were brought by miracles to

believe, since these, as was said above, force and take
away from him free agency in spiritual things. Everything forced in such things, brings itself into the natural
man, and shuts up, as with a door, the spiritual, which
is truly the internal man, and deprives this of all power
of seeing any truth in the light; wherefore afterwards
he reasons concerning spiritual things from the natural
man alone, which sees every thing truly spiritual upside
down. But the reason that miracles were done, before
the coming of the Lord, was, because then the men of
the church were natural, to whom spiritual things, which
are the internals of the church, could not be opened;
for if they had been opened, they would have profaned
them.—TRUE CHRISTIAN RELIGION, 500, 501.

ORDER IN REGENERATION

Before the natural man is conjoined to the spiritual,
or the external man to the internal, it is left to him to
think, whether he is willing that the concupiscences
arising from the love of self and the world, and the considerations by which he had defended them, should be
abolished, and the spiritual or internal man be vested
with dominion;—it is left to him to think thus, to the
intent that he may freely choose what he pleases. When
the natural man without the spiritual thinks on this,
he instantly rejects it, for he loves his concupiscences,
because he loves himself and the world; whence he becomes anxious, and supposes that, if those concupiscences were abolished, there would be no more life remaining with him, for he places his all in the natural
or external man; or he supposes that afterwards he shall
have no self-ability, and that whatever he thinks, wills,
and acts, will flow-in through heaven, thus that he will
no longer be his own master.

When the natural man left to himself is in this state,
he draws himself back, and resists; but when any light
through heaven from the Lord flows into his natural,

he begins to think that it is better that the spiritual man should have dominion, for thereby he can think and will what is good, and thus can come into heaven, which he could not do if the natural were to have rule. And when he thinks that all the angels in the universal heaven are of this character, and that hence they are in ineffable joy, he then enters into combat with the natural man, and at length is willing that it should be made subordinate to the spiritual. In this state the man is placed that is to be regenerated, to the intent that he may freely turn whither he will, and so far as he freely turns in the above direction, so far he is regenerated.—HEAVENLY ARCANA, 5650.

ORDER IN DIVINE OPERATION AND HUMAN CO-OPERATION

The Lord continually withdraws man from evils, so far as man from a free principle is willing to be withdrawn; so far as he can be withdrawn from evils, so far he is drawn by the Lord to good, thus to heaven. So far as man cannot be withdrawn from evils, so far he cannot be drawn by the Lord to good, thus to heaven; for man, so far as he is withdrawn from evils, so far doeth good from the Lord, which good in itself is good, but so far as he is not withdrawn from evils, so far he doeth good from himself, which good in itself hath evil.

Man, by the speech of his mouth, and by the actions of his body, is in the natural world, but by the thoughts of his understanding and by the affections of his will he is in the spiritual world. By the spiritual world is meant both heaven and hell, each distinguished most ordinately into innumerable societies, according to all the varieties of affections and consequent thoughts. In the midst of those societies is man, so tied to them that he cannot exercise in the slightest instance either his thought or will, but together with them, and so together, that if he was to be plucked away from them, or they from him, he would fall down dead, retaining only life in his inmost principle, by which principle he is a man and not a beast, and by which principle he lives to eternity. Man does not know that he is in such inseparable consorts as to life, and the reason why he does not know it is, because he does not discourse with spirits, consequently, he does not know anything concerning that state.

Man from his birth is in the midst of infernal societies, and dilates himself into them, altogether as he dilates the evil affections of his will. The evil affections of the will are all derived from the loves of self and of the world; because those loves turn all things of the mind downwards and outwards, thus to hell, which is beneath, and which is out of themselves, and thereby averts them from the Lord, thus from heaven. The interior also of all things of the human mind, and therewith the interiors of all things of the spirit, are turned downwards when man loves himself above all things; and they are turned upwards when he loves the Lord above all things. It is an actual turning; man of himself turns them downwards, and the Lord from Himself turns them upwards; the reigning love is what turns. Thoughts do not turn the interiors of the mind, except so far as they are derived from the will.

That man may be brought out of hell, and brought into heaven, by the Lord, it is necessary that he should resist hell, that is, evils, as from himself; if he does not resist as from himself, he remains in hell, and hell in him, nor are they separated to eternity.

The Lord alone resists evils with man, because to resist evils with man is of Divine Omnipotence, Divine Omniscience, and Divine Providence. It is of Divine Omnipotence, because to resist one evil is to resist many, and likewise is to resist the hells. Every single evil is conjoined with inumerable evils, and their coherence is like that of the hells with each other, for as evils so the hells, and as the hells so evils, make one, and to resist the hells so conjoined is impossible for any one but the Lord alone. It is of Divine Omniscience, because the Lord alone knows what is the quality of man, and what his evils are, and in what connection they are with other evils, thus in what order they are to be removed, that man may be healed from within, or radically. It is of Divine Providence, lest anything be done contrary to the laws of order, also, that what is done may promote the happiness of man to eternity; for Divine Providence, Divine Omniscience, and Divine Omnipotence, in all things, have respect to what is eternal.—APOCALYPSE EXPLAINED, 1162–65.

SENSUAL ORDER

A man may easily apperceive whether sensual things are in the first place or in the last; if he affirms every thing which the sensual advises or appetites, and endeavours to invalidate every thing which the intellectual dictates, in this case sensual things are in the first place, and the man is carried away by his appetites, and is altogether sensual. Such a man is not far removed from the condition of the irrational animals, which are carried away exactly in the same manner. He is in a worse condition, if he abuses the intellectual or rational faculty to confirm the evils and falses which sensual things advise and appetite. If he does not affirm them, but interiorly sees the deviations thereof into falses, and the excitations thereof to evils, and endeavours to correct those things, and to subject them to the intellectual and will-part of the interior man, in this case sensual things are reduced into order, so that they are in the last place. When they are in the last place, there flows a happy and blessed principle from the interior man into the delights of things sensual, and causes the delights thereof a thousand times to exceed the former delights. The sensual man does not believe that this is the case, because he does not comprehend it; and as he is sensible of no other delight than the sensual, and thinks that there is no higher delight, he regards as of no account the happy and blessed prin-

ciple which is within the delights of sensual things; for
what is unknown to any one, is believed not to be.—
HEAVENLY ARCANA, 5725.

OBSTRUCTIONS TO ORDER

There are two loves, and their lusts which obstruct
the influx of heavenly love from the Lord; for those
loves, whilst they have rule in the interior and external
man, and take possession of it, either reject or suffocate
the heavenly love in its influx, and also pervert and de-
file it, being altogether contrary to such heavenly love.
But in proportion as those loves are removed, heavenly
love, entering by influx from the Lord, begins to appear,
yea, to shine bright in the interior man; and in the same
proportion man begins to see that he is in evil and falsity,
yea, afterwards, that he is in uncleanness and defile-
ment, and, lastly, that this was his proprium. These
are they who are regenerate, with whom those loves are
removed. It may also be apperceived by the unre-
generate, with whom, when the lusts of those loves are
quiescent, (as is the case at times whilst they are in holy
meditation, or whilst their lusts are laid asleep, as happens under great misfortunes, or in times of sickness,
and chiefly at the hour of death,) they apperceive somewhat of heavenly light, and of comfort from it; in consequence of corporeal and worldly things being then laid
asleep, and in a manner dead; but with such there is not
any removal of those lusts, but only a suspension of their
activity, as in sleep; for they instantly relapse into them
on their recovery of their pristine state. . . . It is to be
observed, that there is a continual influx of heavenly
love from the Lord present with man, and that there
is nothing which opposes, obstructs, and incapacitates
man for its reception, but the lusts originating in the
above loves, and the falsities thence derived.—HEAVENLY
ARCANA, 241, 3041.

XII

ALPHA AND OMEGA

Sound reason dictates that all were predestined to heaven, and no one to hell; for all are born men, and from this the image of God is in them. The image of God is in them in that they can understand truth and do good. To be able to understand truth is from the Divine Wisdom, and to be able to do good is from the Divine Love; this power is the image of God, which remains in a sane man, and is not eradicated. It is from this that he is able to become a civil and moral man; and he who is civil and moral can also become spiritual, for the civil and moral is the receptacle of the spiritual.—DIVINE PROVIDENCE, 322.

Heaven is conjunction with the Lord. Man is from creation such that he can be more and more closely conjoined with the Lord. The more closely a man is conjoined with the Lord, the wiser he becomes. The more closely a man is conjoined with the Lord, the happier he becomes. The more closely a man is conjoined with the Lord, the more distinctly he seems to himself as if he were his own, and the more clearly he recognizes that he is the Lord's.—DIVINE PROVIDENCE, 27.

And I saw a new heaven and a new earth: for the first heaven and the first earth were passed away; and there was no more sea.

And I John saw the holy city, new Jerusalem, coming down from God out of heaven, prepared as a bride adorned for her husband.

And I heard a great voice out of heaven saying, Behold, the tabernacle of God is with men, and he will dwell with them, and they shall be his people, and God himself shall be with them, and be their God.

And God shall wipe away all tears from their eyes; and there shall be no more death, neither sorrow, nor crying, neither shall there be any more pain: for the former things are passed away.

And he that sat upon the throne said, Behold, I make all things new. And he said unto me, Write: for these words are true and faithful.

And he said unto me, It is done. I am Alpha and Omega, the beginning and the end. I will give unto him that is athirst of the fountain of the water of life freely.

He that overcometh shall inherit all things; and I will be his God, and he shall be my son.—REVELATION XXI. 1-7.

CPSIA information can be obtained
at www.ICGtesting.com
Printed in the USA
BVHW040026190322
631662BV00006B/584